An overview of FRCS(T examination

Kishore Puthezhath FRCS (Eng)(Tr & Orth)

2022-05-02

About

This is a short monograph detailing how I prepared for the FRCS Tr & Orth examination in the pre-pandemic time. Following the onset of the COVID19 pandemic in 2020, important changes have been incorporated in the examination process, which I will be enlisting in the following sections.

Includes sample SBA/Viva question of A listed topics.

1 FRCS Tr & Orth Application

Here I'll share my personal experience and tips for FRCS (Tr & Orth) application and preparation:

1.1 Application

Evolution of Orthopaedic training examination in UK

The old-style FRCS: Until late 1970s.

MCh(Orth) from the University of Liverpool: Now obsolete

OPTIONAL Specialty Fellowship exam in orthopaedics in 1979.

A new intercollegiate exam was introduced in 1990, which was accepted by all four Royal Colleges.

In 1991 FRCS became a requirement for accreditation.

The four Surgical Royal Colleges (Edinburgh, England, Glasgow & Ireland) in 2015 introduced a new suite of Intercollegiate Fellowship Examinations for the international surgical community.

The JSCFE had parity of standard with the existing UK/Ireland Intercollegiate Fellowship Examinations and was recognised by GMC for Speciality registration until June 2022.

From June 2022, The JSCFE runs in parallel with the UK and Ireland Intercollegiate Specialty Fellowship Examinations but prospective candidates should note that the two suites of examinations are not equivalent.

It is only JCIE Intercollegiate Specialty Examinations that are regulated by the General Medical Council.

The JSCFE is aimed at surgeons in the international community who are about to, or who have recently completed their training and who wish to continue their careers in countries other than the UK or Ireland.

Success in both JSCFE Section 1 and Section 2 will permit affiliation to one of the four Surgical Royal Colleges of Great Britain and Ireland.

With effect from January 2023, the use of the post-nominal ***IntFRCS (College)*** [not FRCS (College)(Tr & Orth)] distinguishes JCIE examination from JSCFE examination.

1.1.1 Examination Pattern

The current International FRCS (Tr & Orth) exam encompasses two sections: Part I is a written exam and Part II the clinical and oral exam. For further information, and to make sure that your information is up to date, I suggest that you carefully review the Intercollegiate Speciality Board website. This is the link.

1.1.1.0.1 Part I

This section consists of two separate papers (a Computer Based Testing-CBT); essentially, a multiple-choice question (MCQ) paper (2 Hours) and an extended matching question (EMQ) paper (2 hours 30 minutes). Part I is generally regarded as the easier section of exam to pass. A number of candidates may be OK learning for an MCQ/EMI paper but be a long way off the standard for a clinical and viva exam.

Format of Section 1 examination changed from 2021

The GMC has approved an alteration to the format of the Section 1 examination. The following format is applicable to all Section 1 examinations from January 2021:

Paper 1 – 120 Single Best [SBA] (2 hours 15 mins)

Paper 2 – 120 Single Best [SBA] (2 hours 15 mins)

How to apply

https://www.jscfe.co.uk is the official website for registering and applying for the examination. It costs £520.00 for Part I application and £1,785.00 for Part II. To apply,

- Applicants must be six years medically qualified
- Applicants must have passed the MRCS examination before applying for JSCFE examination.
- Applicants must have successfully completed CCT/CCST for JCIE examination and a locally recognised surgical training programme for JSCFE examination and are required to provide evidence of having achieved the required standard of a recognised specialist (day one NHS UK/Ireland consultant standard) in the generality of Trauma and Orthopaedic Surgery
- This evidence must consist of three structured references.
- Examination   Attempts: Candidates will have up to a maximum of 7 years to complete the examination process as follows:
  Section 1:Candidates will have a maximum of 4 attempts   with   no   re-entry
  Section 2:Candidates will have a maximum of 4 attempts   with   no   re-entry

2 Part 1

2.1 Preparing for Part I

Like any other thing in life, there are multiple paths for Part I preparation. Rather than enumerating, I would describe what worked out for me. I believe that, at least 5 months of intense preparation is necessary before you can confidently appear for Part I. Focused preparation begins after the successful submission of application. So, before paying the exam fees, make sure that at least 5-6 months are left for the preparation. It is a good first to answer all the Orthobullets questions to get an idea of where you stand. My score was 40%. I bought Miller's Review of Orthopaedics and started learning. I spent nearly 5-6 hours reading Miller/attempting Orthobullets questions. My strategy was to read Miller as much as I can and as quickly as possible so as to revise at-least 3-4 times. My strategy for Orthobullets questions was similar. My target was 150-200 questions per day, with 3-4 revisions before exam. 1 month before the Part I exam, I bought paid questions in the Orthobullets and BMJ OnExamination which I believe, though expensive, gave me an extra edge and confidence.

2.1.1 My Part I preparation in nutshell was

Miller's review of orthopaedics latest edition, page-to-page, 4 revisions

Orthobullets free questions, 3 revisions

Orthobullets paid questions

BMJ OnExamination

Total 5-6 months preparation spending 5-6 hours on an average daily.

2.1.2 Actual Part I exam experience

Just like any other examination in the past, I reached the city 1 day prior to the exam date. I stayed at a decent 4-star hotel which was located at a walkable distance from the Pearson VUE test Centre. My exam was in the afternoon. I woke up at 6 am. My plan was to brush through the entire Miller before noon, which I did. This gave me a fresh confidence. Had a nice meal and I packed some food to the exam hall.

I consciously abstained from reading/talking anything related to exam from there. Luckily I knew no-one in the exam hall, so I could escape to one corner in the waiting area. I read lightly from my Kindle something other than Orthopaedics and relaxed.

An official checked our passport and gave a brief introduction. I kept all my belongings in to a designated locker, including my mobile after switching off. I was escorted to the test area, and after frisking, was given a pen and a paper for rough work and was taken to the CBT console. Total duration of the exam was 5 hours (2 hours SBA, 2 hours 30 minutes EMQ, 30 minutes break in between). During the break, I was allowed to open the locker, take out my packed food and eat from the waiting area. There were no refreshments provided except for drinking water. The topics/questions I could remember are summarised here

2.1.2.1 The paper

My plan was to see all the questions as quickly as possible and mark the sure shot answers. Then I came back and spent some time on questions which demanded some pondering. Then I came back again to reconsider and review the already answered questions. The flagged questions, the answers of which were not known to me were then reviewed and made some educated guesses. Luckily, still I felt as if I had lot of time.

2.1.2.1.1 The result

The result came as an email from the CHAIR, exactly 20 days after the examination. It also included the breakdown of the result. Mean minimum score required to proceed to Part II was 61.46%. My mean score was 73.39%.

3 Part 2

3.1 Preparing for Part II

3.1.1 New Changes upto July 2022

Section 2 is the clinical component consisting of a series of carefully designed and structured interviews- some scenario-based and some centered around volunteers.

The Section 2 JSCFE examinations will be held in pre-selected world-wide host centres and will not involve volunteers.

3.1.2 Clinical examinations

Examination format (from August 2022)

Clinical Intermediate Cases (2 x 15 minutes) Clinical Short Cases (1 x 15 minutes Upper Limb / 1 x 15 minutes Lower Limb)
Volunteers are used for Intermediate Cases. **Clinical scenarios** are used for Short Cases.

JSCFE examination format

Clinical Intermediate Case (1 case will be discussed in 20 minutes)

Clinical Short Cases (4 cases will be discussed in 20 minutes)

No patients will be present. Clinical Scenarios are used for each Case.

3.1.3 Preparation for PART 2

During the 3 weeks waiting period, I made some internet search and made a tentative plan for Part II preparation, in case I could clear the exam. I was equally thinking about mentally preparing myself to resit the Part I (Though I had no clue about alternative preparation method or my ability to stretch beyond the limits of my initial preparation). It later turned out to be good 1 year gap for the preparation.My plan for Part II can be summarised as below.

1. Attend preparatory course
2. Buy clinical and viva study materials
3. Take classes for residents
4. Standardise the clinical examination method See as much patients as I can
5. Make notes for quick revision
6. Combined study

3.1.4 Preparatory course(s)

I stumbled upon and intuitively selected two courses, which turned out to be real gems in due course,

3.1.4.0.1 Postgraduate Orthopaedics Revision course by Postgraduate Orthopaedics

3.1.4.0.2 The FRCS Mentor Network (Offline youtube videos)

3.1.4.0.3 Postgraduate Orthopaedics Revision course by Paul Banaszkiewicz

This is an intense 6 day course covering all the A list/core topics for Part II. I attended the course twice. One in the very beginning of the Part II preparation and another at the end of my preparation to "iron out my technique", just before exam. The course helped in two fronts; first it helped me to develop a systems approach and secondly it grilled in the concept of **"Higher order thinking"**.

3.1.4.0.4 The FRCS Mentor Network (Offline youtube videos)

Shwan and Firas Arnaout are doing wonderful work in preparing candidates through online group. I regularly listened to their youtube uploads, and believe that this really helped me in developing confidence and foresee the real clinical and viva stations. FRCS mentor group some how introduced me to another gem, videos by Quen Tang.

3.1.4.0.5 Quen Tang videos

This introduced me to two important concepts

- Structured answering in viva using A4 sheet of paper and pencil

- Sleek and crisp presentation

3.1.5 Clinical and viva study material

I stuck to these

- Postgraduate Orthopaedics: The Candidate's Guide to the FRCS (Tr & Orth) Examination
- Postgraduate Orthopaedics: Viva Guide for the FRCS (Tr & Orth) Examination
- Examination Techniques in Orthopaedics by Nick Harris, Fazal Ali
- Pictures from revision notes by Joideep Phadnis
- Pictures from Atlas of human anatomy

3.1.6 Combined study

During the last 2-3 months of preparation, I utilised Zoom application for discussions with my friend Praveen C R.

3.1.7 The Clinical and viva

As usual I reached well in advance before the exam, in fact 2 days earlier. I stayed in the same hotel where viva was supposed to be conducted. Unfortunately, I developed allergic rhinitis and was really worried.

3.1.8 Clinicals, Day 1

I felt quite distracted by the rhinitis and the fellow candidates, with lot of speculative discussions in the air both in the hotel and in the exam hall. I tried not to get carried away and keep focused. I had the short cases first and had to be really on my toes and time fled like anything. My performance was pretty average or possibly bad in 2 stations. Luckily the rhinitis did not come in the way.I tried to forget those stations and tried to focus myself before the intermediate case, sitting away from fellow noisy candidates. I practiced structured history taking by writing down individual questions for standard patient interrogation. In the intermediate case station (PLIF patient with foot drop), I felt more confident and was able to control the situation to a large extend.

3.1.9 Viva, Day 2

Viva was in the morning, but I had lot of time with out any distraction before that. I could revise my entire notes before viva. I could remain focused. Only problem was dry cough, which I tried to ignore. All the questions were familiar to me and I controlled the discussion to a great extend except in the basic science station. There I performed rather poorly, but my overall performance was good.

3.1.10 Dress code

Of course there is no dress code for Part I. For the clinicals, the principle is to be bare below the elbow. Tie is not mandatory. But I preferred to wear one with the end tucked into the Light blue shirt. I wore dark blue trousers and black formal shoes. You are expected to wear a suit for the viva. I wore a dark blue one and a white shirt. The board expects you and only you for the examination. This means no need to carry any examination kit.

3.1.11 Result

Result came as an email from the CHAIR, exactly 10 days after the examination. The email just informed me that I have been successful.

4 Books

4.1 Book review

4.1.1 Introduction

We have the entire Orthopaedic knowledge available online through the wonderful platform of Orthobullets . We have got standard textbooks like Campbell's Operative Orthopaedics, Apley's system of Orthopaedics and Fractures and many more. Our teachers are excellent and they teach their experience in orthopaedics passionately. However, the overall pass percentage(starting from 2009) for Part 1 is around 68% and for the Part 2 it is a little below 60%. Theoretically, after forking out more than £ 2ooo, the possibility of yourself passing both parts in a single attempt is around 40%. This is even lower for International examination. Why it is so?There could be many potential reasons.

Here we will try to stick on to only the critical decision of choosing the study materials in the form of textbooks or online resources. The choice of study material is down to individual preference. Some prefer textbooks while others choose to use websites. Two of my friends claim to pass the Part 1 after studying only Orthobullets question. This could be entirely possible, but I cannot understand how. Hence I here-by label them as outliers!

Like anything else in life, choosing the right resource at the right time is critical, if you want to pass an examination like FRCS(Tr&Orth). It is considered a very difficult examination, where the candidates are tested for the **knowledge** and **understanding** of a wide range of orthopaedic problems. Reading "standard" textbooks and journals may not be enough for passing the examination. The most commonly mentioned prerequisites are **higher order thinking**, **communication skill** and **confidence**. Here I would like to review some of the outstanding books and online resources which could be a potential resource(s) for your success.

4.1.2 Useful websites

4.1.2.1 Part 1

4.1.3 www.orthobullets.com

Orthobullet's questions are the first possible starting point for anybody who wants to assess oneself. It will also help you to get into the groove. At this point temptation to memorize the entire Orthobullets by heart is a real risk, which I believe, is better to resist. Orthobullets provide explanations at the end of each of the questions, stick on to that. and you can also monitor your progress easily, and that too for free. Though American in origin, most of the topics on which questions are created seem relevant to British exam.

4.1.4 www.onexamination.com

FRCS(Tr&Orth) If you should attempt Orthbullets in the beginning of your preparation, then there is another little secret. Go through the on examination questions at the end of your preparation. Along with the paid questions of Orthobullets, this little gem will give you some extra edge on that day.

4.1.5 Part 2

www.frcsortho.com

The previous candidate experience given in the website could be a refresher for those who have successfully completed the Part 1 and not yet started serious Part 2 preparation.Whether one should register for the paid questions is doubtful. I coughed up £200 and feel like I have wasted that money, considering the poor quality and seemingly unreliable information given for that hefty sum.Even they have failed to make the website https secured.

YouTube channels:I wont be repeating what I have discussed

4.2 Recommended Text books

From a plethora of expensive Orthopaedic textbooks of varying size, shape and quality, it is difficult to select a perfect book or two. **It is better to acknowledge the fact that the nature of the exam is diverse and there is no quick and easy remedy.**

4.2.1 Miller's Review of Orthopaedics 7th edition.

Coming with a punchy tag line, *go-to certification and recertification review guide for every orthopaedic resident, fellow, and surgeon*, this book divides people in to two-**Those who believe in Miller's review and those who do not!** It's strong point is compactness and intensiveness; same is its weakness. It's basic science, Arthroplasty and Statistics chapters are industry standard. I cleared the Part 1 **studying** mainly(95%) Miller and Orthobullet question bank. If allowed to grade as per FRCS Part 2 marking system, I will give 7/8 for this book when used for **Part 1**. Its usefulness for Part 2 as an exclusive guide is at the best doubtful. I cannot comment on the more recent 8th edition.

4.2.2 Postgraduate Orthopaedics, the candidate's guide and Viva guide

Selection of Part 2 book is relatively simpler. This book series stands apart. I doubt whether you can pass the Part 2 without going through these 2 books. Apart from the top class content, they drill in **higher order thinking** and caters to even more advanced students of orthopaedics. It is impossible to grade this book. **Prof. Paul Banaszkiewicz has done a work of genius.**

4.2.3 Do you have any proof?

Let's try to learn a topic from these two books: **Funnel plot**

Miller's Review 7th edition: The topic is not covered.

4.2.3.1 Postgraduate Orthopaedics:

Both Candidate's guide and the viva guide beautifully discusses the funnel plot. Let me quote a few lines from them.

4.2.3.1.1 Candidates guide

"Funnel plots are used to compare outcomes in groups of different sizes. It was seen in the section on SEM that with increasing sample size the SEM approaches zero; where this does not occur it is likely that some effect is being observed. This can be used to detect ' outliers '*

In outcome studies, such as when comparing mortality rates for different surgical centres or surgeons **Inverted funnel plots can be used to detect publication bias**; the SEM should be larger for studies with smaller sample sizes – If it is not this may indicate publication bias. ....; if there is an effect of the intervention there will be a shift of the data points to the left but there should still be a greater scatter of results for the studies with a larger SEM. The plot on the left shows no such increase in scatter with increasing SEM, suggesting publication bias(two funnel plots are shown)"

4.2.3.1.2 Viva Guide

"This is called a funnel plot which is a simple scatterplot of the treatment effects (RR) estimated from individual studies (horizontal axis) against the precision of the studies represented by standard error (SE). The vertical dotted line shows the estimated combined RR from the meta-analysis. The diagonal dotted lines show the range in which studies might be distributed by chance given the size (and thus precision) of each study. Thus larger (big sample size), more precise (smaller standard error) studies should be closely distributed either side of the pooled effect and smaller studies should be distributed more widely giving the classic inverted symmetrical funnel. If the studies are not distributed randomly (due to sampling error) around the combined RR estimate then some other influence is suggested. The funnel plot shows trials scattered asymmetrically around the pooled RR with smaller trials reporting a greater effect than larger ones. Two possible explanations are: smaller trials of lower methodological quality tend to overestimate true effect; publication bias has led to the smaller negative trials remaining unpublished." You would appreciate the difference the moment you read a lesser book.

4.2.3.1.3 Concise Orthopaedic notes

Recently Firas Arnaout of FRCS Mentor group contacted me and suggested me to read his recently revised book, **Concise Orthopaedic Notes** . He kindly gave me free assess to the digital version. I thank him for the gesture, even though, as a kindle unlimited member, I had already rented and read some chapters of his book before. Authors believe that they have covered the depth and width of knowledge and skills required for the exam and challenge anyone to find an FRCS question that has not been included in the book. This book is a welcome edition and with some hard work, it can even compete with Miller's review to some extent, *for Part 1.*

Let's see what does the book tell us about funnel plot.

- "Performance measuring tool used to measure variations in performance between surgeons and/or centres and identify outliers (Above red line)
- They are scatter plots, with superimposed control limits (typically 2 SD, 3 SD or 4 SD)
- Shows 90-day mortality following hip surgery
- Surgeon/hospital highlighted as orange triangle
- The smaller the size of the sample, the wider the control limits (increased variability).

- As the sample increases the certainty increases and the 'funnel' is formed.
- Progression along horizontal axis means that surgeon/hospital done more cases
- Data within the control limits (between the dotted lines) are consistent with common cause variation or natural variation, whereas those outside these limits indicate unexpected good or bad results (outliers)
- For mortality, it means they done higher risk patients
- Can't identify someone doing very few cases (towards left side of graph) as outlier.
- Progression along vertical axis means surgeon/hospital have had more of the end point (revision or death) deaths.
- Vertical axis figures presented as standardized ratio.
- For mortality - data adjusted to take account of surgeons who operate on more higher-risk or lower-risk patients.
- Surgeons on central (green) horizontal line have had exactly average expected mortality.
- Surgeons either side of green line but below upper red line have level of mortality that is within expected range.
- Surgeons that appear above top red line have mortality rate higher than expected. This is followed by a picture of funnel plot."

After reading this I am more confused than confident

4.3 Adjutants

1. **FRCS Tr & Orth Exam- A guide to clinical and viva by Mansoor   Kassim**
   A straightforward, precise and short guide which is a delight to read. Excellent for Part 2.

2. **Examination technique in Orthopaedics** Harris and Ali's is **the** clinical examination guide for FRCS(Tr&Orth), period

3. **Practice of Paediatric Orthopaedics by Lynn T. Staheli**
   This book is a delight to read. After passing the exam, I am still reading it very often. Short, precise and insightful.

4. **Orthopaedic surgical approaches by Mark D. Miller**
   While the anatomic approach Hoppenfeld is the standard textbook for studying exposures, this book is refreshingly new.

5. **Orthopaedic notes by Joideep Phadnis** If you dig enough in the World Wide Web, you will get this book for free. The pictures are first class and the notes are extensive.

6. **Basic Orthopaedic Sciences by Manoj Ramachandran** No comments.

7. **Netter's Concise Orthopaedic Anatomy by Jon C Thompson** Small book, concise and useful to some extend

4.4 Conclusions

- There is no single book/resource that can guarantee a pass for you.
- Select your 'jab' early and take the full dose.
- **Revision is the key. Hence, grab the information from reliable resources, understand it and make your own notes   ,   especially   after   Part   1**

5 FRCS (TR &ORTH) QUESTIONS

5.1 SBA/EMQ

- Supracondylar fracture 4 seconds cap filling , full stomach.

- Supracondylar fracture not able to flex index finger.

- Supracondylar fracture, compartment syndrome , structure involved: brachial artery

- Lateral condyle pinning open, not able to give bye bye 7 year old

- Green colour to cement: chlorophyll

- Prevent cement polymerisation

- Proximal stimulation motor ganglia: f wave

- Muscle fibrillation: COMP

- DELAY across elbow: latency

- Ultrasound

- Push-up is what type of exercise

- Lengthening followed by contraction

- Muscle fibre in Achilles tendon

- Irregularly arranged 1 and 2 collagen seen in

- Multifascicular with vascular supply and type 4 collagen

- Finger drop with wrist in flexion and radial deviation

- Structure retracted to see cervical vertebrae anterior

- Structure torn and retracted inferiority in c spine anterior sx

- Structure damaged above c3 anterior sx

- Anterior knee pain TKA normal Xray, Cause

- Instabily CR TKA, on climbing staircase

- 20 degree extension lag after resurfacing

- Pelvic metastasis not responding to rt

- Wide excision and prosthetic replacement done in : thyroid, TX, breast, humerus, trochanter, greater trochanter, lesser trochanter

- Damage control Orthopaedics, marker: 11 6

- Candilever failure cause:

- Charnley hip failure, M/C in :OA, RA, tip medial or lateral

- No wear after 10 years THA

- Not good in females THA

- Moderate wear with ductility THA

- DEXA true

- Differentiate cortical and trabicular osteoporosis

- Attach with sharpy fibers

- Resusitated , better then hypotension fluid under diaphragm, pelvic binder: 2 more crystalloid or abdl CT or laparotomy

- Hammer toe with stiffness

- Mallet finger

- Flexible claw toes treatment

- Abducor hallucis weakness nerve

- Plane for mid tibia posterior

- Proximal fibula plane

- Originate from mid fibula

- Transverse arch maintained by

- Structure accompanied by sciatic nerve

- Variably present in ilioinguinal approach

- Plane between TFL and gluteal medius

- Splitting gluteus medius approach

- ASA 3 70 shopping neck of femur fracture treatment

- Gustello periosteal stripping no flap

- Scaphoid 6 week conservative , ballottment and pain after that what to do

- Rheumatoid cannot flex thumb

- Rheumatoid caput ulae

- Spiral fracture humerus radial nerve palsy treatment

- Structure damaged in dislocation young

- Subtalar evasion and tibia IR in

- Eccentric contraction to prevent lateral lurch

- Muscle that concentrically contracture to extend hip

- Eccentrically contracting muscle stance phase

- X-ray showing navicular osteonecrosis : treatment

- Photo extensor muscle wasting thumb

- Photo 30 degree abd muscle testing

- Radial head dislocated congenital, treatment

- Picture showing cervical myelopathy with loss of lordosis treatment

- Buford complex

- Buford complex ligament

- Ligament preventing inferior translation neutral addiction

- TSA anterior dislocation cause

- Vessel damaged in carpal tunnel release

- Zone 2 injury little finger fdp lost no tenodesis sign for fds

- Flexar tenosynovitis

- Click on getting up from chair rugby player elbow

- Proximal femur fraCture deformity

- Most common cause intoeing gait 10 year old

- Change made in the departmental study: audit

- Rails in CVA patient house, type of study: cross sectional

- Reamed vs unreamed: RCT

- Post op blood transfusion m/c cause

- 2 years after scaphoid no arthritis treatment

- Trapezectomy in rheumatoid

- Plexus upper

- TOS in adult

- Gamella superior nerve supply

- Gait muscles

- Sacroiliac joint nerve involved

- Dial test

- High tibia osteotomy in varus knee

- CP patient with pain no power head out GMFCS CLASS

- Subtrochanteric fracture failure cause

- P value

- Mean and standard deviation

- Triplane fracture treatment

- 7 year old lamping investigation

- Double size , torsion strength pin

- Double size bending strength plate

- Plane volar Henry

- Clinicals

- Short cases

- High ulnar nerve palsy with elbow FFD

- Short lady with polyarthritis, neck stiffness and deformities

- Soft tissue swelling ankle

- Young OA knee, Opposite side with scar of HTO

- Intermediate

- Old gentleman with neurogenic claudication, scar of PLIFF, foot drop

5.2 Viva

5.2.1 Basic science

Infection control in ward

Knee Anatomy (atlas picture)

Chondrosarcoma shoulder

Xxx

Xxx

xxx

5.2.2 Trauma

Lisfranc

Epiphyseal injury Distal Femur

Leg compartment

Facet joint dislocation

Xxx

xxx

5.2.3 Adult pathology

DDH THA

Parsonage Turner Syndrome

Compartment syndrome

Xxx

Xxx

xxx

5.2.4 Paeds and Hand

Supracondylar fracture

LLD

DDH

Boutonniere

Tendon repair

Xxx

6 BOAST guidelines

It is desirable to know the common BOAST guidelines, which is also considered ad quoting the literature, making one eligible for 7 or 8 in the Viva/Clinicals.

Guidelines

Printed in Great Britain
by Amazon